LOW HISTAMINE COOKBOOK FOR SENIORS

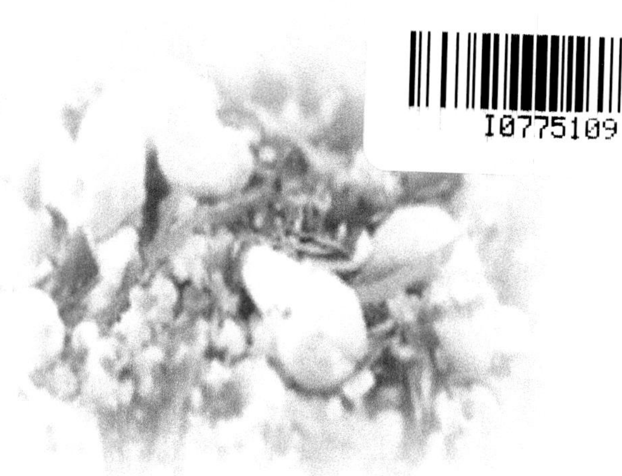

Quick and Easy Recipes to Reverse Histamine Intolerance and Relieve your Symptoms.

David T. Salcedo

TABLE OF CONTENTS

INTRODUCTION

Meet Emma, a retired schoolteacher who enjoys culinary experimentation. Emma learned about her own histamine sensitivity later in life, and it became a conundrum she was motivated to solve. Inspired by her experience, she set out to produce a cookbook customized to the preferences and needs of her fellow seniors.

Her little kitchen became a hive of exploration, filled with the tantalizing fragrances of carefully chosen ingredients. Emma collected a number of like-minded friends, each with their own story about discovering histamine sensitivity, and they formed a culinary community that enthusiastically accepted the challenge.

As they stirred pots and pans and exchanged stories of culinary triumphs and tribulations, the seniors discovered the thrill of creating meals that not only satiated their taste senses but also supported their bodies. The kitchen became a hub of laughing, companionship, and the occasional friendly debate about the ideal seasoning.

The cookbook they prepared reflected their common experiences. It was more than just a compilation of recipes; it was a guide to seniors' low histamine dining options. Each page conveyed a tale, from the scented breakfasts that greeted the day to the warm dinners that ended it. The cookbook was a treasure trove of culinary knowledge.

The elders discovered that they not only mastered the technique of low histamine cooking, but also enjoyed sharing their knowledge with others. They held cookery lessons, and the town's younger generations enthusiastically took up their elders' wisdom. The aroma of foods boiling on stovetops became a symbol of unification, uniting generations via a shared appreciation of delicious cuisine.

Word traveled beyond their area, and elderly from nearby communities sought their advice. The cookbook served as an inspiration for folks dealing with histamine intolerance. Emma and her pals, who were formerly satisfied in their tiny hamlet, had unintentionally become culinary teachers, causing a ripple effect of flavor, health, and community.

In the end, the Low Histamine Cookbook for Seniors was more than simply a collection of recipes; it was a monument to the fortitude of a group of determined people who transformed a dietary problem into a culinary adventure. As the seniors gathered around a table laden with histamine-friendly pleasures, they realized that their tale, recorded in the language of food, would continue to inspire others to taste life's flavors, no matter what obstacles they faced.

WHAT IS HISTAMINE SENSITIVITY

Histamine sensitivity, also known as histamine intolerance, is a disorder in which the body fails to adequately metabolize histamine, resulting in a buildup of the substance. Histamine is a neurotransmitter and immune system mediator that regulates several body activities. When histamine levels surpass the body's ability to break them down, it can cause a variety of symptoms and pain.

Causes of Histamine sensitivity

Enzyme Deficiency: Low levels of DAO and HNMT, enzymes that break down histamine, can lead to sensitivity.

Gut Health Issues: Conditions such as SIBO, leaky gut syndrome, and gastrointestinal infections can disrupt histamine metabolism.

Dietary Factors: Consuming histamine-rich meals (e.g., aged cheeses, fermented items), histamine-releasing foods (e.g., citrus fruits, tomatoes), and foods that inhibit DAO can cause sensitivity.

Drugs: Some drugs, including NSAIDs, antipsychotics, and proton pump inhibitors, might disrupt histamine breakdown.

Genetic Predisposition: Certain genetic variants can reduce enzyme function, increasing susceptibility to histamine sensitivity.

Symptoms of Histamine Sensitivity

Digestive Symptoms

- Abdominal pain

- Bloating

- Diarrhea or constipation

Skin Reactions

- Hives

- Eczema

- Itching

Respiratory Symptoms

- Sneezing

- Nasal congestion

- Asthma-like symptoms

Neurological Symptoms

- Headaches, including migraines.

- Dizziness

- Anxiety

Cardiovascular Symptoms

- Fluctuations in blood pressure

- Rapid heart rate

Treatment

Low Histamine Diet

Eliminating high-histamine foods and those that trigger histamine release is the basic method. This could include avoiding fermented foods, certain dairy items, and alcohol.

Supplements

Take DAO supplements before meals to improve histamine breakdown in the digestive tract.

Probiotics

Probiotics may improve gut health by reducing histamine-producing microorganisms.

Antihistamines

Prescribing antihistamines may alleviate symptoms, although their effectiveness varies.

Preventive Measures

Dietary Awareness

Identifying and avoiding trigger foods is essential. Keeping a food journal can help you discover specific triggers.

Stress Management

Stress might worsen symptoms. Meditation, yoga, and deep breathing are all effective techniques.

Environmental Considerations

Minimizing exposure to allergens and pollution can reduce histamine levels.

Gradual Reintroduction

With guidance from a healthcare practitioner, gradually reintroduction of foods as symptoms improves.

THE SIGNIFICANCE OF A LOW HISTAMINE DIET FOR SENIORS

As people age, their bodies change in a variety of ways, including alterations in metabolic processes and the efficiency of organ functioning. For some elders, regulating histamine levels is an important part of preserving general health and well-being. A reduced histamine diet is becoming acknowledged as a crucial component in treating histamine sensitivity in seniors, with several physical and mental health benefits.

Understanding Histamine Sensitivity in Seniors

Histamine sensitivity arises when the body's ability to break down histamine is impaired, resulting in an excess of the chemical in the bloodstream. Seniors may be more susceptible to histamine sensitivity as their digestive enzymes and gut health alter with age. Common symptoms include stomach troubles, skin sensitivities, breathing problems, headaches, and others.

Impact on Senior Health

Digestive Comfort

Histamine sensitivity can worsen age-related digestive difficulties, including bloating, abdominal pain, and irregular bowel movements. A low-histamine diet can help with these symptoms.

Skin and Respiratory Health

Seniors may experience eczema, nasal congestion, and asthma-like symptoms. Managing histamine consumption through diet can help to improve skin and respiratory health.

Cognitive Well-Being

Histamine plays a role in neurotransmission and can impact cognitive functions. When adopting a low histamine diet, seniors may notice increased mental clarity as well as fewer headaches and dizziness.

Cardiovascular Stability

Symptoms of histamine sensitivity, such as blood pressure fluctuations and high heart rate, might be risky, particularly for elderly individuals. A low-histamine diet may help to maintain cardiovascular stability.

Improved Energy Levels

Seniors frequently struggle with weariness and low energy levels. A reduced histamine diet, by reducing histamine-induced reactions, may improve general energy and vitality.

HOW TO IMPLEMENT A LOW HISTAMINE DIET FOR SENIORS

Selecting Senior-Friendly Foods

This diet prioritizes fresh, unprocessed foods, making it ideal for seniors seeking to maintain or improve their nutritional intake. Fresh fruits and vegetables, lean proteins, and certain grains can be included.

Avoiding High-Histamine Foods

Seniors should avoid histamine-rich meals including aged cheeses, cured meats, and fermented items, as well as those that trigger histamine release, such tomatoes and alcohol.

Customizing Based on Health Conditions

A low histamine diet can be adapted for seniors with specific dietary limitations or recommendations depending on their health needs.

COMMON HEALTH ISSUES IN SENIORS EXACERBATED BY HISTAMINE

Gastrointestinal Disorders

Histamine Impact: with histamine sensitivity may report worsening symptoms of gastrointestinal diseases such IBS, gastritis, or GERD.

Symptoms: Excess histamine can worsen symptoms such as abdominal pain, bloating, indigestion, and bowel changes

Neurological Conditions

Histamine Impact: Imbalanced histamine levels can increase symptoms of migraines, tension headaches, and other cognitive issues.

Symptoms: Seniors with histamine sensitivity may experience more frequent and intense headaches, migraines, and cognitive problems such as brain fog.

Dermatological Issues

Histamine Impact: Seniors with histamine sensitivity may experience worsened skin diseases such eczema, psoriasis, and chronic itching due to the inflammatory response caused by histamine.

Symptoms: Symptoms include increased itching, redness, and inflammation, resulting in discomfort and poor skin health.

Respiratory Disorders

Histamine Impact: Histamine can worsen symptoms of asthma, COPD, and other respiratory conditions in seniors.

Symptoms: Seniors may have worsening coughing, wheezing, and shortness of breath, making it difficult to maintain their respiratory health properly.

Cardiovascular Concerns

Histamine Impact: Fluctuations in blood pressure and heart rate, common symptoms of histamine sensitivity, might exacerbate pre-existing cardiovascular disorders in seniors, such as hypertension or arrhythmia.

Symptoms: Histamine's impact on blood vessel dilatation and heart rate may raise the risk of cardiovascular events for seniors.

Autoimmune Disorders

Histamine Impact: Histamine can affect autoimmune illnesses such as rheumatoid arthritis and lupus, causing inflammation and joint pain in seniors.

Symptoms: Seniors with histamine sensitivity and autoimmune illnesses may have worsening joint pain, edema, and stiffness.

FOOD TO EAT AND FOOD TO AVOID

Foods to Eat

1. **Fresh Meats**

   - Chicken

   - Turkey

   - Fresh fish (excluding high-histamine varieties like tuna, mackerel, and sardines)

2. **Fresh Fruits**

   - Apples

   - Pears

   - Berries (strawberries, blueberries, raspberries)

   - Mangoes

3. **Fresh Vegetables**

   - Leafy greens (spinach, kale, lettuce)

   - Zucchini

   - Broccoli

   - Carrots

   - Sweet potatoes

4. **Dairy Alternatives**

   - Coconut milk

- Almond milk

- Rice milk

5. **Grains**

    - Rice (white or brown)

    - Quinoa

    - Oats (certified gluten-free)

6. **Fresh Herbs**

    - Basil

    - Parsley

    - Cilantro

    - Thyme

7. **Cooking Oils**

    - Olive oil

    - Coconut oil

8. **Beverages**

    - Water

    - Herbal teas (non-citrus)

    - Green tea

Foods to Avoid

1. **Fermented Foods**
   - Sauerkraut
   - Kimchi
   - Pickles

2. **Aged Cheeses**
   - Parmesan
   - Cheddar
   - Gouda

3. **Processed Meats**
   - Salami
   - Pepperoni
   - Bacon

4. **Certain Seafood**
   - Tuna
   - Mackerel
   - Sardines

5. **Citrus Fruits**
   - Oranges
   - Lemons

- Grapefruits

6. **Tomatoes and Tomato Products**

   - Tomatoes

   - Tomato sauces

7. **Certain Vegetables**

   - Eggplants

   - Avocados

   - Spinach (in large quantities)

8. **Certain Nuts**

   - Walnuts

   - Cashews

   - Peanuts

9. **Processed and Packaged Foods**

   - Ready-made sauces

   - Packaged snacks with additives and preservatives

10. **Alcoholic Beverages**

    - Wine

    - Beer

    - Certain spirits

CHAPTER 1

Breakfast Recipes

1. Quinoa Breakfast Bowl

Ingredients

- 1 cup cooked quinoa

- 1/2 cup fresh blueberries

- 1 tablespoon chia seeds

- 1 tablespoon pumpkin seeds

- 1 teaspoon honey (optional)

Mode of Preparation

1. Mix cooked quinoa with fresh blueberries, chia seeds, and pumpkin seeds.

2. Drizzle with honey for sweetness (optional).

3. Serve warm.

Nutritional Information

- Calories: 300

- Protein: 10g

- Fiber: 8g

- Healthy Fats: 7g

Serving Size: 1 bowl

Preparation Time: 15 minutes

2. Smoked Salmon Avocado Toast

Ingredients

- 1 slice low histamine bread

- 50g smoked salmon

- 1/2 avocado, sliced

- Fresh dill for garnish

Mode of Preparation:

1. Toast the bread.

2. Top with smoked salmon and sliced avocado.

3. Garnish with fresh dill.

Nutritional Information

- Calories: 250

- Protein: 15g

- Fiber: 7g

- Healthy Fats: 15g

Serving Size: 1 toast

Preparation Time: 10 minutes

3. Sweet Potato Hash with Eggs
Ingredients

- 1 medium sweet potato, grated

- 2 eggs

- 1 tablespoon olive oil

- Fresh parsley for garnish

Mode of Preparation:

1. Sauté grated sweet potato in olive oil until tender.

2. Make wells in the sweet potato and crack eggs into them.

3. Cover and cook until eggs are done.

4. Garnish with fresh parsley.

Nutritional Information

- Calories: 320

- Protein: 14g

- Fiber: 6g

- Healthy Fats: 18g

Serving Size: 1 serving

Preparation Time: 20 minutes

4. Spinach and Mushroom Omelette

Ingredients

- 2 eggs

- 1/2 cup fresh spinach, chopped

- 1/4 cup mushrooms, sliced

- 1 tablespoon olive oil

- Salt and pepper to taste

Mode of Preparation:

1. Sauté mushrooms and spinach in olive oil until wilted.

2. Whisk eggs and pour over the vegetables.

3. Cook until eggs are set. Season with salt and pepper.

Nutritional Information

- Calories: 220

- Protein: 14g

- Fiber: 3g

- Healthy Fats: 15g

Serving Size: 1 omelette

Preparation Time: 15 minutes

5. Chia Pudding with Berries

Ingredients

- 2 tablespoons chia seeds

- 1 cup almond milk

- 1/2 cup mixed berries

- 1 teaspoon vanilla extract

Mode of Preparation

1. Mix chia seeds, almond milk, and vanilla extract. Refrigerate overnight.

2. Top with mixed berries before serving.

Nutritional Information:

- Calories: 180

- Protein: 6g

- Fiber: 10g

- Healthy Fats: 8g

Serving Size: 1 cup

Preparation Time: Overnight + 5 minutes

6. Greek Yogurt Parfait

Ingredients

- 1/2 cup low histamine Greek yogurt

- 1/4 cup granola (low histamine)

- 1/2 cup fresh kiwi slices

- 1 tablespoon honey (optional)

Mode of Preparation

1. Layer Greek yogurt, granola, and kiwi in a glass.

2. Drizzle with honey for sweetness (optional).

Nutritional Information

- Calories: 280

- Protein: 12g

- Fiber: 5g

- Healthy Fats: 8g

Serving Size: 1 parfait

Preparation Time: 10 minutes

7. Quinoa and Berry Breakfast Parfait

Ingredients

- 1/2 cup cooked quinoa

- 1/2 cup low histamine Greek yogurt

- 1/4 cup mixed berries (blueberries, strawberries)

- 1 tablespoon slivered almonds

- 1 teaspoon honey (optional)

Mode of Preparation

1. Layer cooked quinoa, Greek yogurt, and mixed berries in a glass.

2. Repeat the layers.

3. Top with slivered almonds and drizzle with honey for sweetness (optional).

Nutritional Information

- Calories: 280

- Protein: 12g

- Fiber: 5g

- Healthy Fats: 7g

Serving Size: 1 parfait

Preparation Time: 15 minutes

8. Buckwheat Pancakes with Berries

Ingredients

- 1/2 cup buckwheat flour

- 1/2 cup almond milk

- 1 egg

- 1/2 teaspoon baking powder

- Mixed berries for topping

Mode of Preparation

1. Mix buckwheat flour, almond milk, egg, and baking powder.

2. Cook pancakes on a non-stick pan.

3. Top with mixed berries.

Nutritional Information

- Calories: 220

- Protein: 8g

- Fiber: 5g

- Healthy Fats: 6g

Serving Size: 2 pancakes

Preparation Time: 15 minutes

9. Coconut and Banana Muffins

Ingredients

- 1 cup coconut flour

- 2 ripe bananas, mashed

- 1/4 cup coconut oil

- 3 eggs

- 1/2 teaspoon baking soda

Mode of Preparation

1. Mix coconut flour, mashed bananas, melted coconut oil, eggs, and baking soda.

2. Pour into muffin cups and bake until golden.

Nutritional Information

- Calories: 180

- Protein: 4g

- Fiber: 6g

- Healthy Fats: 12g

Serving Size: 1 muffin

Preparation Time: 20 minutes

10. Rice Cake with Almond Butter and Banana

Ingredients

- 1 rice cake (low histamine)

- 1 tablespoon almond butter

- 1/2 banana, sliced

- Cinnamon for garnish

Mode of Preparation

1. Spread almond butter on the rice cake.

2. Top with banana slices and a sprinkle of cinnamon.

Nutritional Information

- Calories: 180

- Protein: 4g

- Fiber: 3g

- Healthy Fats: 8g

Serving Size: 1 rice cake

Preparation Time: 5 minutes

CHAPTER 2

Lunch recipes

1. Grilled Chicken Salad Bowl
Ingredients

- Grilled chicken breast

- Mixed salad greens (lettuce, spinach, arugula)

- Cherry tomatoes

- Cucumber

- Olive oil and lemon dressing

Preparation

- Grill chicken breast and slice.

- Toss salad greens, cherry tomatoes, and cucumber.

- Drizzle with olive oil and lemon dressing.

Nutritional Information

- Calories: 300

- Protein: 25g

- Fat: 15g

- Carbohydrates: 18g

- Fiber: 5g

Serving Size: 1 bowl

Preparation Time: 20 minutes

2. Quinoa and Vegetable Stir-Fry
Ingredients

- Quinoa

- Broccoli

- Bell peppers

- Carrots

- Coconut aminos (low-histamine soy sauce alternative)

Preparation

- Cook quinoa according to package instructions.
- Stir-fry vegetables in coconut aminos.
- Combine quinoa and stir-fried vegetables.

Nutritional Information

- Calories: 250
- Protein: 10g
- Fat: 8g
- Carbohydrates: 40g
- Fiber: 6g

Serving Size: 1 cup

Preparation Time: 25 minutes

3. Salmon and Avocado Lettuce Wraps

Ingredients

- Grilled salmon

- Avocado slices

- Bibb lettuce leaves

- Dill and lemon for seasoning

Preparation

- Grill salmon and break into flakes.
- Place salmon and avocado slices on lettuce leaves.
- Season with dill and a squeeze of lemon.

Nutritional Information

- Calories: 280
- Protein: 20g
- Fat: 18g
- Carbohydrates: 8g
- Fiber: 5g

Serving Size: 2 wraps

Preparation Time: 15 minutes

4. Turkey and Sweet Potato Hash

Ingredients

- Ground turkey

- Sweet potatoes, diced

- Spinach

- Olive oil

- Paprika and salt for seasoning

Preparation

- Brown ground turkey in olive oil.

- Add diced sweet potatoes and cook until tender.

- Mix in spinach and season with paprika and salt.

Nutritional Information

- Calories: 320

- Protein: 22g

- Fat: 12g

- Carbohydrates: 28g

- Fiber: 5g

Serving Size: 1 cup

Preparation Time: 30 minutes

5. Zucchini Noodles with Pesto and Shrimp

Ingredients

- Zucchini noodles

- Shrimp, peeled and deveined

- Homemade basil pesto (olive oil, basil, pine nuts, garlic)

Preparation

- Sauté shrimp until cooked.

- Spiralize zucchini into noodles.

- Toss zucchini noodles with shrimp and pesto.

Nutritional Information

- Calories: 260

- Protein: 18g

- Fat: 16g

- Carbohydrates: 10g

- Fiber: 3g

Serving Size: 1.5 cups

Preparation Time: 20 minutes

6. Egg Salad Lettuce Wraps
Ingredients

- Hard-boiled eggs, chopped

- Celery, finely chopped

- Green onions, sliced

- Mayonnaise (homemade or store-bought)

Preparation

- Combine chopped eggs, celery, and green onions.

- Mix in mayonnaise until well combined.

- Spoon into lettuce leaves for wraps.

Nutritional Information

- Calories: 220

- Protein: 12g

- Fat: 18g

- Carbohydrates: 3g

- Fiber: 1g

Serving Size: 3 wraps

Preparation Time: 15 minutes

7. Baked Cod with Lemon and Herbs

Ingredients

- Cod fillets

- Fresh herbs (parsley, thyme)

- Lemon slices

- Olive oil

Preparation

- Cod fillets should be placed on a baking sheet.

- It should be drizzled with olive oil and sprinkle with herbs.

- Top with lemon slices and bake until fish is flaky.

Nutritional Information

- Calories: 180

- Protein: 25g

- Fat: 8g

- Carbohydrates: 2g

- Fiber: 0g

Serving Size: 1 fillet

Preparation Time: 25 minutes

8. Lentil and Vegetable Soup

Ingredients

- Green lentils

- Carrots, diced

- Celery, chopped

- Low-histamine vegetable broth

- Fresh parsley for garnish

Preparation

- Combine lentils, carrots, and celery in a pot with vegetable broth.

- Simmer until lentils are cooked through.

- Garnish with fresh parsley before serving.

Nutritional Information

- Calories: 220

- Protein: 15g

- Fat: 1g

- Carbohydrates: 40g

- Fiber: 10g

Serving Size: 2 cups

Preparation Time: 40 minutes

9. Spinach and Turkey Stuffed Bell Peppers

Ingredients

- Ground turkey

- Bell peppers, halved

- Spinach, chopped

- Tomato sauce (low-histamine)

Preparation

- Brown ground turkey and mix with chopped spinach.

- Stuff bell peppers with the turkey and spinach mixture.

- Top with low-histamine tomato sauce and bake until peppers are tender.

Nutritional Information

- Calories: 290

- Protein: 25g

- Fat: 12g

- Carbohydrates: 20g

- Fiber: 6g

Serving Size: 2 halves

Preparation Time: 35 minutes

10. Roasted Vegetable and Chicken Quinoa Bowl

Ingredients

- Roasted chicken breast

- Mixed roasted vegetables (zucchini, bell peppers, cherry tomatoes)

- Cooked quinoa

- Olive oil and lemon dressing

Preparation

- Chicken and vegetables should be roasted in the oven.

- Mix roasted chicken and vegetables with cooked quinoa.

- Drizzle with olive oil and lemon dressing.

Nutritional Information

- Calories: 320

- Protein: 25g

- Fat: 10g

- Carbohydrates: 30g

- Fiber: 5g

Serving Size: 1 bowl

Preparation Time: 30 minutes

CHAPTER 3

Dinner Recipes

1. Grilled Salmon with Lemon Herb Sauce

Ingredients

- 4 salmon fillets

- 2 tablespoons olive oil

- 1 lemon (juiced)

- 1 teaspoon dried oregano

- Salt and pepper to taste

Mode of Preparation

1. Preheat the grill.

2. Season salmon fillets with salt, pepper, and oregano.

3. Grill salmon for 4-5 minutes per side or until cooked through.

4. In a small bowl, mix olive oil and lemon juice for the sauce.

5. Drizzle the lemon herb sauce over grilled salmon.

Nutritional Information

- Calories: 350

- Protein: 30g

- Carbohydrates: 2g

- Fat: 25g

- Fiber: 0g

Serving Size: 1 fillet

Preparation Time: 20 minutes

2. Turkey and Vegetable Stir-Fry

Ingredients

- 1 lb ground turkey

- 2 cups broccoli florets

- 1 bell pepper (sliced)

- 1 zucchini (sliced)

- 2 tablespoons coconut oil

- 2 tablespoons low-sodium soy sauce

Mode of Preparation

1. In a pan, brown ground turkey in coconut oil.

2. Add vegetables and stir-fry until tender.

3. Add soy sauce and continue cooking for 2-3 minutes.

Nutritional Information

- Calories: 300

- Protein: 25g

- Carbohydrates: 10g

- Fat: 18g

- Fiber: 4g

Serving Size: 1 cup

Preparation Time: 25 minutes

3. Chicken and Vegetable Skewers

Ingredients

- 1 lb chicken breast (cubed)

- 1 zucchini (sliced)

- 1 red onion (sliced)

- 2 tablespoons olive oil

- 1 teaspoon dried thyme

- Salt and pepper to taste

Mode of Preparation

1. Preheat the grill.

2. Thread chicken, zucchini, and onion onto skewers.

3. Mix olive oil, thyme, salt, and pepper for marinade.

4. Grill skewers for 10-12 minutes, turning occasionally.

Nutritional Information

- Calories: 280

- Protein: 30g

- Carbohydrates: 5g

- Fat: 15g

- Fiber: 2g

Serving Size: 2 skewers

Preparation Time: 30 minutes

4. Quinoa and Roasted Vegetable Salad

Ingredients

- 1 cup quinoa (cooked)

- 1 cup cherry tomatoes (halved)

- 1 cucumber (diced)

- 1 bell pepper (diced)

- 2 tablespoons balsamic vinaigrette

- Fresh basil leaves for garnish

Mode of Preparation

1. In a bowl, combine quinoa, cherry tomatoes, cucumber, and bell pepper.

2. Drizzle with balsamic vinaigrette and toss gently.

3. Garnish with fresh basil leaves.

Nutritional Information

- Calories: 220

- Protein: 8g

- Carbohydrates: 40g

- Fat: 4g

- Fiber: 6g

Serving Size: 1 cup

Preparation Time: 15 minutes

5. Baked Cod with Herbed Potatoes

Ingredients

- 4 cod fillets

- 4 cups baby potatoes (halved)

- 2 tablespoons olive oil

- 1 teaspoon dried rosemary

- Salt and pepper to taste

Mode of Preparation

1. Preheat the oven.

2. Season cod fillets with salt, pepper, and rosemary.

3. Toss potatoes in olive oil and season with salt.

4. Place cod and potatoes on a baking sheet and bake for 20-25 minutes.

Nutritional Information

- Calories: 290

- Protein: 30g

- Carbohydrates: 20g

- Fat: 10g

- Fiber: 3g

Serving Size: 1 fillet with potatoes

Preparation Time: 30 minutes

6. Vegetarian Stuffed Bell Peppers

Ingredients:

- 4 bell peppers (halved)

- 1 cup cooked quinoa

- Black beans (drained and rinsed) of 1 Can

- 1 cup corn kernels

- 1 cup diced tomatoes

- 1 teaspoon cumin

- 1 teaspoon chili powder

Mode of Preparation

1. Preheat the oven.

2. In a bowl, mix quinoa, black beans, corn, tomatoes, cumin, and chili powder.

3. Stuff bell peppers with the mixture.

4. Bake for 25-30 minutes.

Nutritional Information

- Calories: 280

- Protein: 12g

- Carbohydrates: 50g

- Fat: 3g

- Fiber: 10g

Serving Size: 2 halves

Preparation Time: 40 minutes

7. Salmon and Asparagus Foil Packets

Ingredients

- 4 salmon fillets

- 2 bunches asparagus

- 2 tablespoons lemon juice

- 2 tablespoons olive oil

- Fresh dill for garnish

Mode of Preparation

1. Preheat the oven.

2. Place salmon fillets on sheets of foil.

3. Arrange asparagus around salmon.

4. Drizzle with lemon juice and olive oil, then seal the foil packets.

5. Bake for 15-20 minutes.

Nutritional Information

- Calories: 320

- Protein: 30g

- Carbohydrates: 8g

- Fat: 20g

- Fiber: 4g

Serving Size: 1 packet

Preparation Time: 25 minutes

8. Mushroom and Spinach Omelette

Ingredients:

- 4 eggs

- 1 cup sliced mushrooms

- 1 cup fresh spinach

- 2 tablespoons olive oil

- Salt and pepper to taste

Mode of Preparation

1. Eggs should be beaten in a bowl and season with salt and pepper.

2. In a skillet, sauté mushrooms and spinach in olive oil.

3. Pour beaten eggs over vegetables and cook until set.

Nutritional Information

- Calories: 250

- Protein: 15g

- Carbohydrates: 5g

- Fat: 20g

- Fiber: 2g

Serving Size: 1 omelette

Preparation Time: 15 minutes

CHAPTER 4

Snacks recipes

1. Avocado and Cucumber Sushi Rolls

Ingredients

- Nori sheets

- Avocado, sliced

- Cucumber, julienned

- Cooked quinoa (cooled)

- Tamari sauce (low-sodium)

Mode of Preparation

1. Nori sheet should be placed on a sushi rolling mat.

2. Spread a thin layer of cooked quinoa on the nori sheet.

3. Arrange avocado and cucumber slices along the center.

4. Roll the sushi tightly, using water to seal the edge.

5. Slice into bite-sized pieces and serve with low-sodium tamari sauce.

Nutritional Information

- Calories: 150

- Protein: 3g

- Fat: 9g

- Carbohydrates: 15g

- Fiber: 4g

Serving Size: 4 rolls

Preparation Time: 20 minutes

2. Baked Sweet Potato Chips

Ingredients

- Sweet potatoes, thinly sliced

- Olive oil

- Sea salt

- Paprika (optional)

Mode of Preparation

1. Preheat the oven to 375°F (190°C).

2. Toss sweet potato slices with olive oil and sprinkle with sea salt (and paprika if desired).

3. Slices should be placed on a baking sheet in a single layer.

4. Bake for 15-20 minutes or until crispy.

5. Allow to cool before serving.

Nutritional Information

- Calories: 120

- Protein: 2g

- Fat: 5g

- Carbohydrates: 18g

- Fiber: 3g

Serving Size: 1 cup

Preparation Time: 25 minutes

3. Hummus and Veggie Sticks

Ingredients

- Low histamine hummus (store-bought or homemade)

- Carrot sticks

- Cucumber spears

- Bell pepper strips

Mode of Preparation

1. Arrange veggie sticks on a plate.

2. Serve with a side of low histamine hummus for dipping.

Nutritional Information

- Calories: 100

- Protein: 3g

- Fat: 5g

- Carbohydrates: 12g

- Fiber: 4g

Serving Size: 1 cup veggies + 2 tbsp hummus

Preparation Time: 10 minutes

4. Quinoa Salad Cups

Ingredients:

- Cooked and cooled quinoa

- Cherry tomatoes, halved

- Fresh basil, chopped

- Olive oil

- Balsamic vinegar

- Salt and pepper to taste

Mode of Preparation

1. In a bowl, mix quinoa, cherry tomatoes, and basil.

2. It should be drizzled with olive oil and balsamic vinegar.

3. Season with salt and pepper.

4. Spoon the mixture into small cups for serving.

Nutritional Information

- Calories: 180

- Protein: 5g

- Fat: 7g

- Carbohydrates: 24g

- Fiber: 3g

Serving Size: 1 cup

Preparation Time: 15 minutes

5. Rice Cake with Smoked Salmon and Dill

Ingredients

- Rice cakes

- Smoked salmon

- Fresh dill, chopped

- Lemon slices

Mode of Preparation

1. Top each rice cake with smoked salmon.

2. Garnish with chopped dill and a squeeze of lemon.

Nutritional Information

- Calories: 120

- Protein: 8g

- Fat: 5g

- Carbohydrates: 15g

- Fiber: 1g

Serving Size: 2 rice cakes

Preparation Time: 10 minutes

6. Stuffed Bell Peppers with Tuna Salad

Ingredients

- Bell peppers, halved and seeds removed

- Canned tuna, drained

- Greek yogurt (low-fat)

- Celery, finely chopped

- Green onions, sliced

- Dill, chopped

- Salt and pepper to taste

Mode of Preparation

1. In a bowl, mix tuna, Greek yogurt, celery, green onions, and dill.

2. Season with salt and pepper.

3. Spoon the tuna salad into halved bell peppers.

Nutritional Information

- Calories: 150

- Protein: 15g

- Fat: 5g

- Carbohydrates: 10g

- Fiber: 2g

Serving Size: 2 pepper halves

Preparation Time: 15 minutes

7. Apple and Almond Butter Slices

Ingredients

- Apples, thinly sliced

- Almond butter (low histamine)

Mode of Preparation

1. Spread almond butter on apple slices.

2. Arrange on a plate and serve.

Nutritional Information

- Calories: 130

- Protein: 3g

- Fat: 8g

- Carbohydrates: 15g

- Fiber: 3g

Serving Size: 1 medium apple + 2 tbsp almond butter

Preparation Time: 5 minutes

8. Baked Kale Chips

Ingredients

- Fresh kale, washed and dried

- Olive oil

- Nutritional yeast (optional)

- Sea salt

Mode of Preparation

1. Preheat the oven to 350°F (175°C).

2. Toss kale with olive oil, nutritional yeast, and sea salt.

3. Arrange on a baking sheet and bake until crispy.

4. Allow to cool before serving.

Nutritional Information

- Calories: 80

- Protein: 5g

- Fat: 4g

- Carbohydrates: 10g

- Fiber: 3g

Serving Size: 1 cup

Preparation Time: 15 minutes

9. Greek Yogurt Parfait with Low-Histamine Fruits

Ingredients

- Greek yogurt (low-fat)

- Pineapple, diced

- Mango, diced

- Kiwi, sliced

- Chopped mint leaves

Mode of Preparation

1. In a glass, layer Greek yogurt with diced pineapple, mango, and kiwi.

2. Repeat the layers.

3. Top with chopped mint leaves.

Nutritional Information

- Calories: 180

- Protein: 15g

- Fat: 3g

- Carbohydrates: 28g

- Fiber: 4g

Serving Size: 1 cup

Preparation Time: 10 minutes

CHAPTER 5

Smoothies

1. Berry Bliss Smoothie

Ingredients

- 1 cup fresh blueberries

- 1 cup strawberries (hulled)

- 1 ripe banana

- 1 cup coconut milk (low histamine)

- 1 tablespoon chia seeds

Mode of Preparation

1. Blend all the ingredients until smooth.

2. Pour into a glass and garnish with additional berries if desired.

Nutritional Information

- Calories: 250

- Protein: 4g

- Fat: 12g

- Carbohydrates: 35g

- Fiber: 9g

Serving Size: 1 smoothie

Preparation Time: 5 minutes

2. Cucumber Mint Cooler

Ingredients

- 1 cucumber (peeled and sliced)

- 1 cup honeydew melon chunks

- 1/4 cup fresh mint leaves

- 1 cup coconut water (low histamine)

- Ice cubes

Mode of Preparation

1. Combine cucumber, honeydew melon, mint, and coconut water in a blender.

2. Blend until smooth, add ice cubes, and blend again.

Nutritional Information

- Calories: 80

- Protein: 2g

- Fat: 1g

- Carbohydrates: 18g

- Fiber: 3g

Serving Size: 1 smoothie

Preparation Time: 7 minutes

3. Green Goddess Delight
Ingredients

- 1 cup spinach leaves

- 1/2 avocado

- 1/2 cup pineapple chunks

- 1 cup almond milk (low histamine)

- 1 tablespoon flaxseeds

Mode of Preparation

1. Blend spinach, avocado, pineapple, almond milk, and flaxseeds until creamy.

2. Pour into a glass and enjoy.

Nutritional Information

- Calories: 220

- Protein: 5g

- Fat: 14g

- Carbohydrates: 25g

- Fiber: 8g

Serving Size: 1 smoothie

Preparation Time: 6 minutes

4. Coconut-Berry Medley
Ingredients

- 1/2 cup raspberries

- 1/2 cup blackberries

- 1/2 cup coconut yogurt (low histamine)

- 1 tablespoon hemp seeds

- 1/2 cup coconut water

Mode of Preparation:

1. Blend raspberries, blackberries, coconut yogurt, hemp seeds, and coconut water until smooth.

2. Serve in a chilled glass.

Nutritional Information

- Calories: 180

- Protein: 4g

- Fat: 9g

- Carbohydrates: 22g

- Fiber: 8g

Serving Size: 1 smoothie

Preparation Time: 5 minutes

5. Tropical Turmeric Twist

Ingredients

- 1/2 cup mango chunks

- 1/2 cup pineapple chunks

- 1 teaspoon turmeric powder

- 1 cup rice milk (low histamine)

- 1 tablespoon chia seeds

Mode of Preparation

1. Blend mango, pineapple, turmeric, rice milk, and chia seeds until smooth.

2. Pour into a glass and enjoy this immune-boosting delight.

Nutritional Information

- Calories: 220

- Protein: 5g

- Fat: 4g

- Carbohydrates: 40g

- Fiber: 8g

Serving Size: 1 smoothie

Preparation Time: 6 minutes

6. Peachy Keen Smoothie

Ingredients

- 1 cup peaches (sliced)

- 1/2 cup cucumber (peeled and sliced)

- 1/2 cup coconut milk (low histamine)

- 1 tablespoon sunflower seeds

- Ice cubes

Mode of Preparation

1. Blend peaches, cucumber, coconut milk, sunflower seeds, and ice cubes until creamy.

2. Pour into a glass and savor the refreshing taste.

Nutritional Information

- Calories: 180

- Protein: 4g

- Fat: 11g

- Carbohydrates: 22g

- Fiber: 4g

Serving Size: 1 smoothie

Preparation Time: 5 minutes

7. Vanilla Almond Dream

Ingredients

- 1/2 cup sliced almonds

- 1/2 teaspoon vanilla extract

- 1 banana

- 1 cup almond milk (low histamine)

- Ice cubes

Mode of Preparation

1. Blend sliced almonds, vanilla extract, banana, almond milk, and ice cubes until smooth.

2. Pour into a glass, and enjoy the nutty goodness.

Nutritional Information

- Calories: 260

- Protein: 6g

- Fat: 18g

- Carbohydrates: 24g

- Fiber: 6g

Serving Size: 1 smoothie

Preparation Time: 6 minutes

8. Melon Mint Marvel

Ingredients

- 1 cup cantaloupe chunks

- 1/2 cup honeydew melon chunks

- 1 tablespoon fresh mint leaves

- 1 cup coconut water (low histamine)

- Ice cubes

Mode of Preparation

1. Blend cantaloupe, honeydew melon, mint, coconut water, and ice cubes until smooth.

2. Pour into a glass and garnish with mint leaves.

Nutritional Information

- Calories: 90

- Protein: 2g

- Fat: 1g

- Carbohydrates: 22g

- Fiber: 2g

Serving Size: 1 smoothie

Preparation Time: 5 minutes

9. Cherry Almond Delight

Ingredients

- 1/2 cup cherries (pitted)

- 1/2 cup almond butter

- 1 cup rice milk (low histamine)

- 1 tablespoon chia seeds

- Ice cubes

Mode of Preparation:

1. Blend cherries, almond butter, rice milk, chia seeds, and ice cubes until creamy.

2. Pour into a glass and enjoy the rich, nutty flavor.

Nutritional Information

- Calories: 320

- Protein: 7g

- Fat: 24g

- Carbohydrates: 26g

- Fiber: 8g

Serving Size: 1 smoothie

Preparation Time: 7 minutes

10. Mango-Coconut Elixir

Ingredients

- 1 cup mango chunks
- 1/2 cup coconut cream (low histamine)
- 1/2 cup pineapple chunks
- 1 tablespoon shredded coconut
- 1 cup coconut water

Mode of Preparation

1. Blend mango, coconut cream, pineapple, shredded coconut, and coconut water until smooth.
2. Pour into a glass and garnish with additional shredded coconut.

Nutritional Information

- Calories: 280
- Protein: 3g
- Fat: 21g
- Carbohydrates: 25g
- Fiber: 4g

Serving Size: 1 smoothie

Preparation Time: 6 minutes

CHAPTER 6

7 Days Meal Plan

Day 1

Breakfast- Quinoa Breakfast Bowl

Lunch- Grilled Chicken Salad Bowl

Dinner- Grilled Salmon with Lemon Herb Sauce

Day 2

Breakfast- Smoked Salmon Avocado Toast

Lunch- Quinoa and Vegetable Stir-Fry

Dinner- Turkey and Vegetable Stir-Fry

Day 3

Breakfast- Sweet Potato Hash with Eggs

Lunch- Salmon and Avocado Lettuce Wraps

Dinner- Chicken and Vegetable Skewers

Day 4

Breakfast- Spinach and Mushroom Omelette

Lunch- Turkey and Sweet Potato Hash

Dinner- Quinoa and Roasted Vegetable Salad

Day 5

Breakfast- Chia Pudding with Berries

Lunch- Zucchini Noodles with Pesto and Shrimp

Dinner- Baked Cod with Herbed Potatoes

Day 6

Breakfast- Greek Yogurt Parfait

Lunch- Egg Salad Lettuce Wraps

Dinner- Vegetarian Stuffed Bell Peppers

Day 7

Breakfast- Quinoa and Berry Breakfast Parfait

Lunch- Baked Cod with Lemon and Herbs

Dinner- Salmon and Asparagus Foil Packets

CHAPTER 7

Conclusion

Low Histamine Cookbook for Seniors has been a rich tapestry of flavors, healthful choices, and shared stories. Through the chapters, we have ventured into the intricate realm of histamine sensitivity, discovering not only the challenges it presents but also the empowering possibilities that lie within a low histamine diet.

This book has been crafted with the intention of providing seniors and their loved ones with a compass for navigating the complexities of histamine sensitivity. From the foundational understanding of histamine and its impact on aging bodies to the practical kitchen wisdom needed to create delicious low histamine meals, we have embarked on a path that intertwines health, joy, and community.

The recipes shared within these pages are not just culinary creations; they are invitations to savor life, to celebrate the diversity of flavors, and to foster a connection with one's well-being. From the refreshing Berry Bliss Smoothie to the comforting Peachy Keen Smoothie, each recipe has been designed not only to meet the dietary needs of seniors but also to elevate the pleasure of dining.

Histamine sensitivity, a unique challenge faced by many seniors, has been met here with understanding, respect, and creative solutions. The kitchen, once a realm of potential frustration, has become a space for exploration and mastery. Our seniors, through their stories and shared wisdom, have illuminated the transformative power of embracing a low histamine lifestyle.

As we close the chapter on this cookbook, let it serve as a constant companion for seniors on their journey to health and vibrancy. Let it be a source of inspiration for families, caregivers, and friends who seek to create meals that nourish both the body and the soul. In each recipe, in each story, we find the resilience of the human spirit and the profound impact that mindful, low histamine living can have on the golden years.

May the scent of these dishes linger in your kitchens, the flavors dance on your taste buds, and the shared moments around the table become cherished memories. For, in the world of low histamine cooking, we have discovered not just a dietary choice but a celebration of life, a celebration that continues long after the last page is turned. Here's to health, here's to joy, and here's to savoring every delicious moment on this nourishing journey.

THANKS FOR READING